RON KNESS

Anti-Aging Secrets

Tips and Techniques to Keep You Looking Young

ISBN: 9798714618925

Published by:

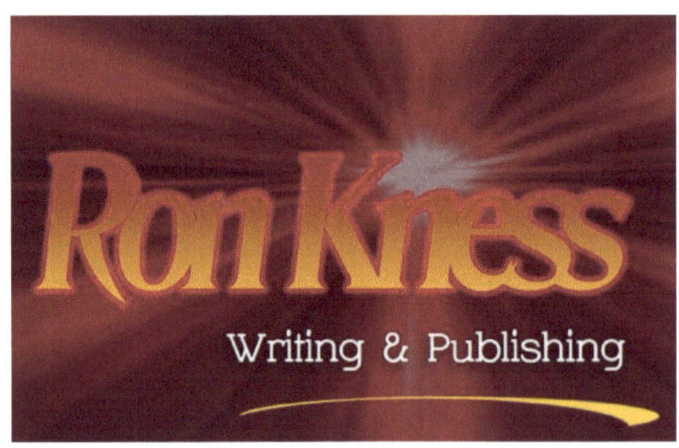

https://ronknesswriting.com

Ron Kness

Queen Creek, AZ

United States of America

For

Healthy Lifestyle Newsletter

https://healthylifestylenewsletter.com

Disclaimer

This publication is for informational purposes only and is not intended as medical advice. Medical advice should always be obtained from a qualified medical professional for any health conditions or symptoms associated with them.

Every possible effort has been made in preparing and researching this material. We make no warranties with respect to the accuracy, applicability of its contents or any omissions.

See your healthcare professional before starting any diet, health or exercise program!

Contents

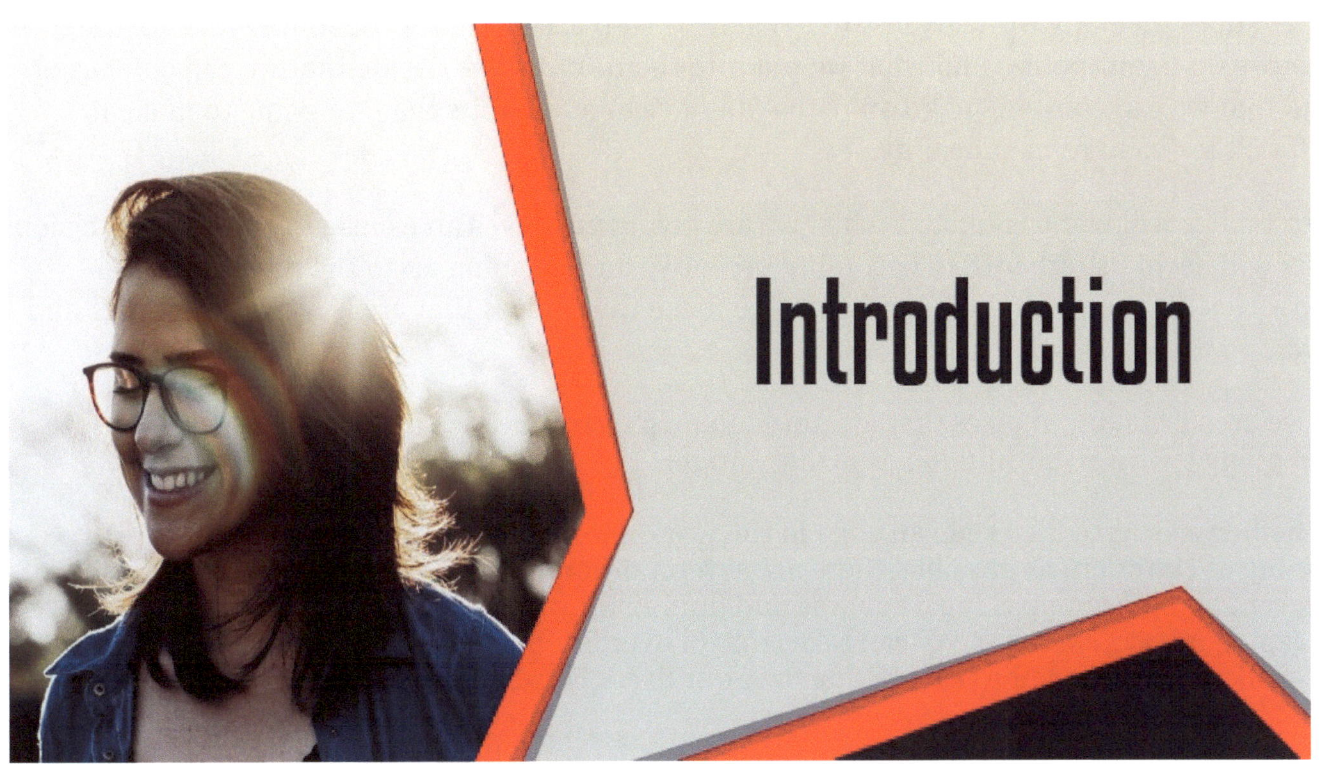

Introduction

For centuries, humans have been obsessed with beauty and youth. We have tried everything from practices we still use today, to some off the wall things that might make one cringe in order to maintain a youthful appearance. With the technology that we have at our disposal now, looking and feeling great is almost down to a science! Even now, scientists are uncovering new tips and tricks to maintaining a youthful appearance that will help us to stay confident and enhance our lives.

While the saying is true that beauty is only skin deep, many people find that maintaining a youthful air is important to keep going on with our routines. The working world is competitive in more ways than one, and it also helps us to stay confident with our friends and partners if we can manage to look younger than our age. It is one of the best compliments one can receive, and this book will help you to uncover several anti-aging hacks that will help you to stay at the top of your game.

The most important thing about focusing our lives on anti-aging is the fact that we are doing everything we can do within our power to view our bodies as machines that are either going to work in our favor or against it. So, when does the body work mostly in our favor? When we supply it with the vital components that it needs to stay at its peak form. Our bodies will work in our favor when we are getting the essential vitamins and nutrients, it will work in our favor when we are drinking enough water, and it will work in our favor when we are exercising.

When does the body work against us? When we stop accepting responsibility for the things that we do to our bodies and what we put into them. When we decide that we can cut corners and that we can continue to go on paths full of vices and habits that are going to make it difficult for us to remain healthy.

Our bodies will work against us when we are giving ourselves an excuse to make bad decisions that will harm us rather than becoming proactive and stepping up to the plate to give ourselves the reason and the motivation to make the choices that are best for our bodies and lives.

If we aren't making choices that are going to help us to embrace a youthful life, then we are not going to live a youthful life. It is that simple.

Whether your goal is to keep an edge in the working world or simply to make sure you are feeling as confident as possible, there are several different things that one can implement to prevent aging from marking its course and diminishing our confidence. We don't have to accept aging at face value! We can take control over our bodies and lives and do everything possible to prevent aging from taking over our lives. This book will show you how!

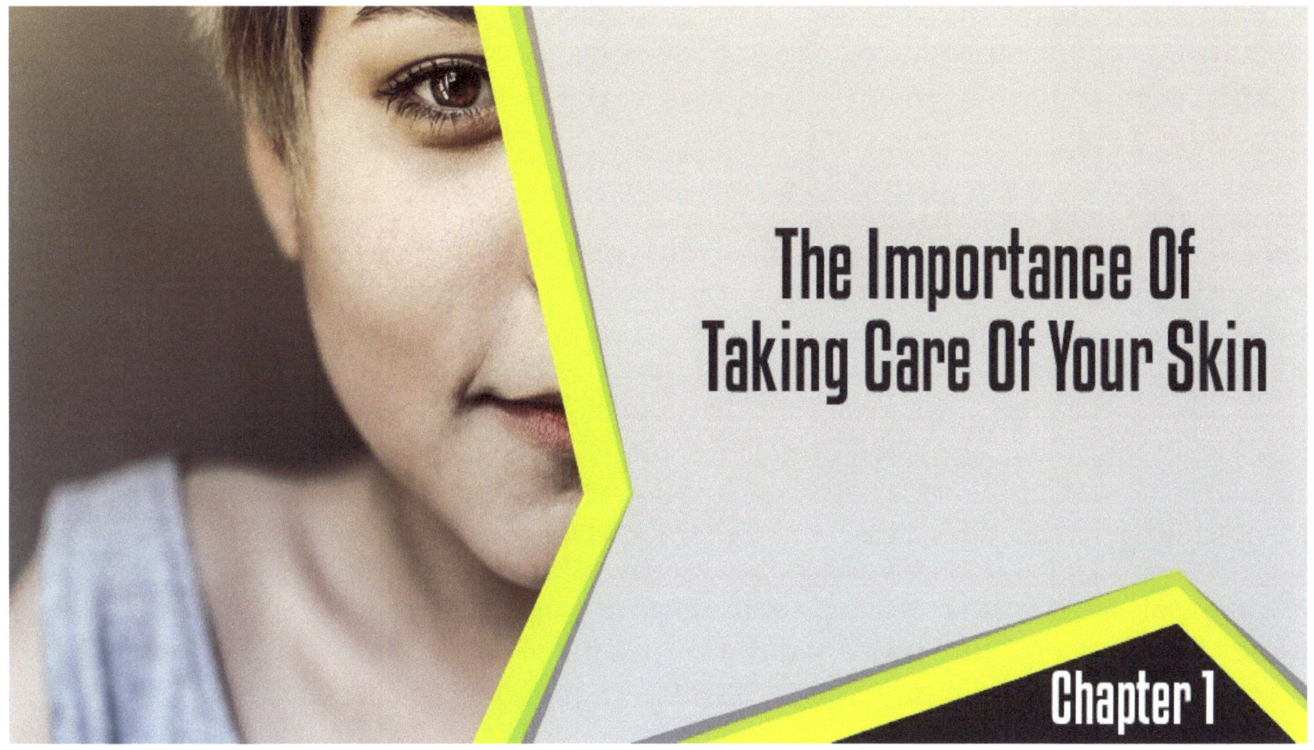

The Importance of Taking Care of Your Skin

When most people think of anti-aging, most of the time what they really want is to make sure that their skin does not show the typical wear and tear that naturally come with growing older. Over time, we often develop habits that make our bodies suffer and eventually we begin to see the results of these poor choices. Fortunately, there are many ways that we can begin to address the bad habits that can cause our skin to look more aged than we are comfortable with. This book will cover these anti-aging hacks in the chapters to come!

The first and foremost of these tips, however, is to do everything possible to take care of your skin and keep it hydrated. If you are not using a good skincare regime now, then it is something to seriously consider for the future. Our skin is what shows the appearance of age, probably more than most other things besides perhaps gray hair … but you can change that at least temporarily!

If you want to have the appearance of youth, what you do and don't do for your skin will really make a difference! Everything that we do has a consequence. If we aren't taking care of our bodies to the best possible extent, then ultimately there will be negative consequences for that. Make sure the consequences that you manifest are the most positive possible!

Our skin is made up of three especially important layers. The external layer is called the epidermis, and contains the protein keratin, which is what eventually continues to grow as our skin cells die and are removed in flakes. It also contains Lagerhans cells, which are a preventative measure our bodies take to ward away bacteria and viruses, along with other things that could ultimately end up making us sick. Our skin insulates us, protects us from water and intense temperatures, and keeps our inner workings safe from sun damage.

It also gives the brain signals through our nerve endings when everything is operating fully. Ultimately, it is one of the most important organs in our body (although it can easily be argued that *every* organ in our body is pretty important!)

The layer of skin below the epidermis is called the dermis and it is also very important. It is more to do with the way things work beneath the surface, such as with the temperature regulation by controlling our blood flow. For example, when it's cold outside, our skin will constrict the flow of our blood, while when it is hot, it actually allows the blood to circulate more quickly so that heat can escape through the surface of our skin.

Our bodies can cool themselves using natural thermodynamic methods, including sweating. However, when we sweat it releases toxins from our bodies that can stay trapped on the skin unless we deal with them quickly. That is why it is so important to keep our skin clean, especially if we want to reduce signs of aging!

Knowing the importance of our skin and how it works can be a vital element in preventing aging from showing up on it. When we understand just how important skin care really is in our daily regimen and caring for our bodies in general to help us get ahead of aging before it's too late, then we will have the tools at our disposal to live a life with the vitality of youth and the confidence to match it! This book will show you how.

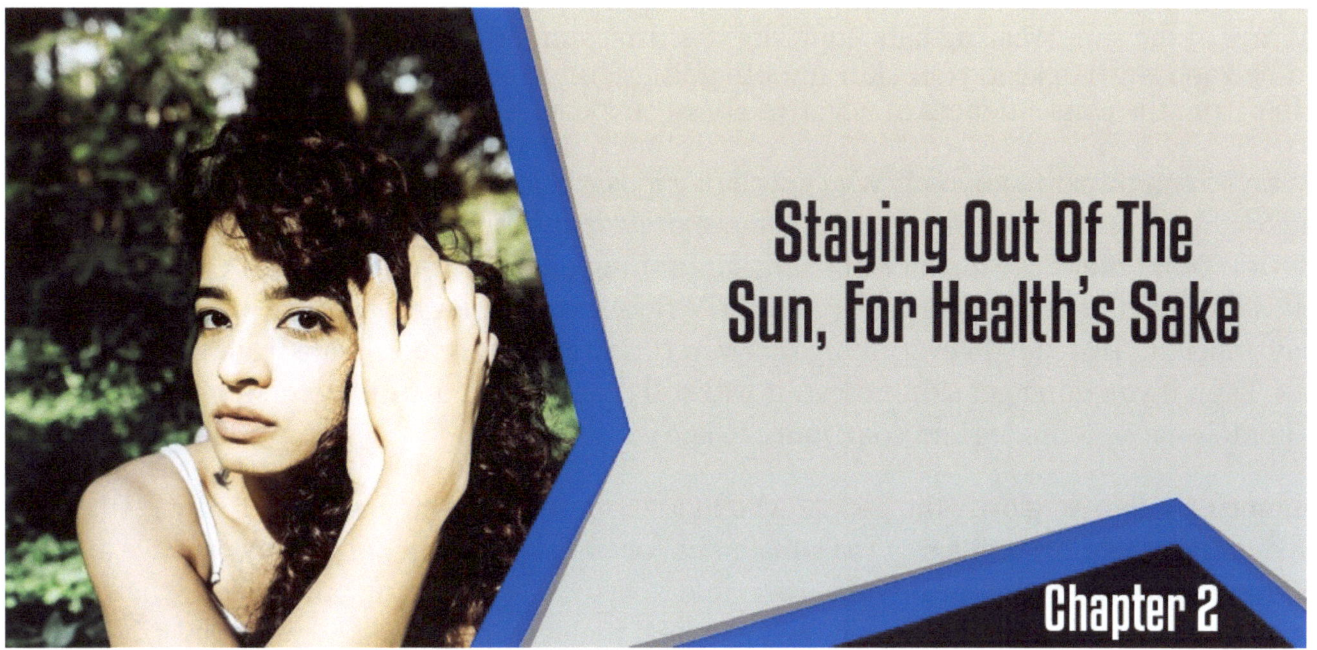

Staying Out of the Sun, for Health's Sake

Many, many people go through life feeling the pressure to look a certain way to feel confident and be accepted by their peers. We want to be attractive, youthful, and confident, and a lot of people find that one of the aesthetics they thrive for is to be tan.

Tanning is a natural process that a lot of people in the Western world have succumbed to encouraging. Sitting out in the sun, rubbing oils on the body so that the sun's rays are attracted to our skin to give it that pleasing, darkened glow, is something so common that it's almost bizarre to consider that it could be harmful.

Unfortunately, the UV rays from the sun's rays can actually cause damage to the skin and cause wrinkles. It can also, over time, cause skin cancer. The negative effects are enhanced greatly if you end up getting sunburnt frequently. This can dry out your skin and cause untold damage to it that can present itself as you age in the form of wrinkles and other blemishes.

When you do get sunburnt, it is important to deal with it immediately. Using things like aloe-vera cream will help you to heal your skin and keep it hydrated despite the damage that has already been done. It will help to do some damage control and provide some relief from the pain of the sunburn as well.

Overall, it is incredibly important to make sure that you are smart about your sun exposure. You want to keep your skin hydrated whether you are in the sun a lot or not, but to prevent wrinkles and dryness, making sure to moisturize becomes even more important. When you go outside, you could try to make sure that you only do so during hours when the suns rays are not as extreme in temperature.

Another thing that you can do is to wear clothing that will protect your body from the harmful UV rays of the sun. Wearing hats, long sleeve shirts, sunglasses, and even carrying a parasol, can be good ways to keep your skin smooth and pristine and prevent yourself from having to suffer from the consequences of negative UV ray exposure.

UV rays are a threat to anybody who gets sun exposure. It is difficult to predict when or how one might get cancer, but skin cancer is more prevalent in those who spend a lot of time out in the sun. Don't make the mistake of using suntanning oil over sunscreen. Don't purposefully expose yourself to tanning beds or natural UV rays for a temporary attempt at glowing and beautiful skin. Instead, do everything that you can to keep your body safe from the harmful rays. Even if you don't get skin cancer, it will still damage and dry out your skin and could ultimately cause wrinkles and contribute to age spots.

Our society tends to glorify the people who look vibrant and tanned without really getting into the details about how damaging the sun can be for our skin. It is a dangerous practice and we will have more long-term beauty if we are able to avoid overexposing ourselves to the sun's rays. Instead of spending money on trying to heal the damage caused by years of sun overexposure, do yourself a favor and prevent it, starting now!

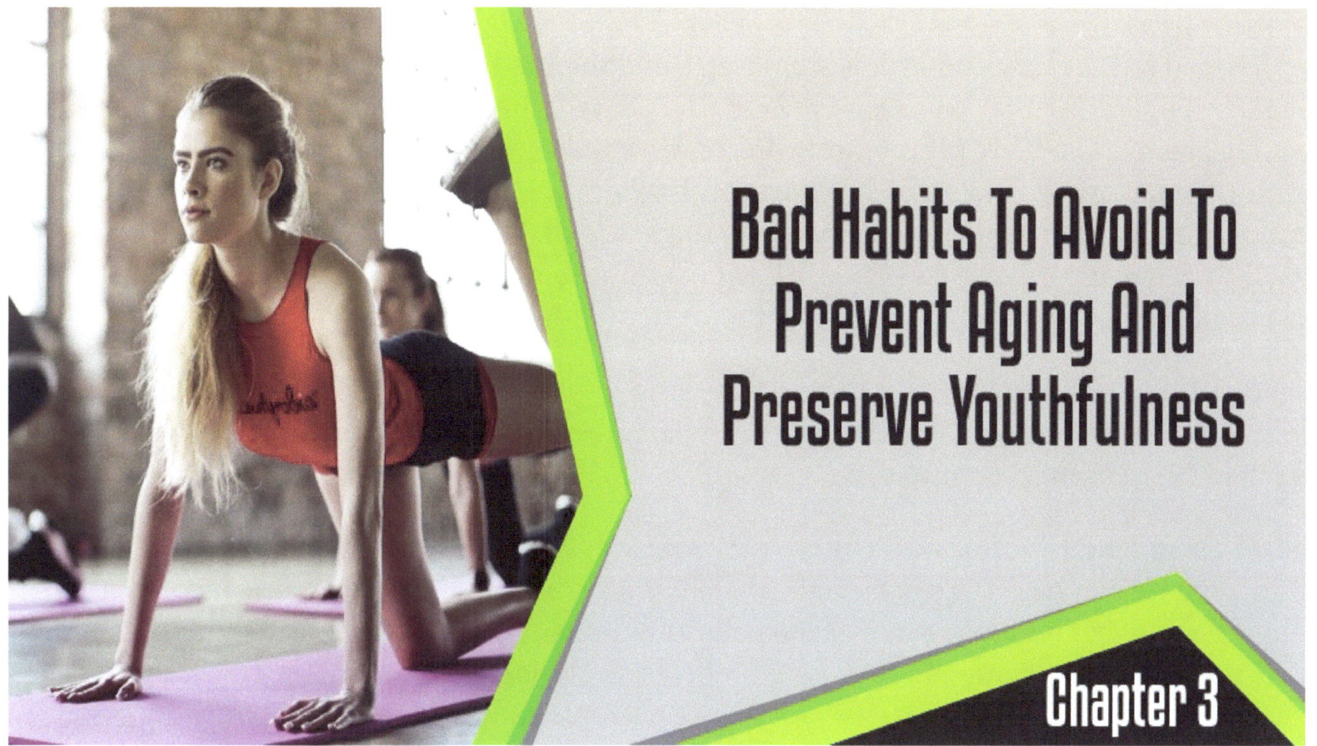

Bad Habits to Avoid to Prevent Aging and Preserve Youthfulness

A lot of us have habits that we perform daily without even thinking twice about it. We may not even think of them as bad habits and simply functions that we perform to go about our days. However, did you know that rubbing your eyes is actually considered dangerous to your skin, especially for those who are concerned about the effects that aging can have on their appearance?

Well, it's true! When we rub our eyes regularly, it can actually cause the damage to the skin around our eyes. This is because it is so thin there that when we rub it, we can easily damage the blood vessels surrounding it. This can lead to decreased blood flow in one of the most sensitive areas on our body and a place that is highly prone to showing the effects of aging on the body.

It can have several different consequences, including a darkened effect around the eyes, or the thickening of the skin around the eyes as it works to consistently repair itself after our thoughtless habits. It can even lead to a lackluster effect that decreases the vibrancy of one of the most captivating parts of our bodies! It's best to avoid rubbing our eyes if at all possible because we don't want to help our bodies age faster than it is necessary!

If you have been prone to rubbing your eyes in the past, have no fear. While it can be true that our past habits can affect us in the present moment, the sooner we address our bad habits and do away with them, the faster we can begin preventing any further damage from occurring. Knowledge truly is power! Especially when we use it wisely.

Another bad habit to try and kick is smoking. Smoking has been known for its negative health effects, but one thing that you aren't necessarily going to hear much about is the way that smoking can age the body prematurely. When we smoke, it takes oxygen away from our cells and can even cause wrinkles around the mouth where we begin to habitually inhale. It causes nicotine stains on the teeth, and sometimes fingers, and it can cause heart and lung problems as well. It can even affect your bones. All things that we want to try and strengthen as we age because of how naturally they become difficult to maintain over time!

Because of the lack of circulation in the body, smokers tend to have colder extremities, such as hands and feet, and may tend to appear to be paler, or have odd coloring in the skin because the blood isn't circulating properly.

Smokers also tend to suffer with baggy and droopy eyes far more so than non-smokers. The skin in general can begin to sag because the chemicals in cigarette smoke are very destructive to the skin and can break down collagen cells and damage our skin's natural elasticity. This can affect everything from our arms to our chests. Smoking can even affect our eyes themselves, causing a higher likelihood of the development of cataracts. These can impair the vision and can generally be dealt with surgically.

Smokers also tend to have more age spots than nonsmokers. Age spots aren't the worst thing in the world, but they can certainly make us look a little bit older than we may truly be. Smokers and people who spend a lot of time exposed to the sun are the most likely to develop age spots.

Something else that isn't mentioned very frequently when it comes to the ways that smoking can make us appear older and decrease our appearance of youthfulness is the fact that people who smoke a lot are far more likely to begin experiencing hair loss. Smoking can thin the hair and excel people predispositions toward balding to experience it at a higher rate.

However, when you quit smoking, your body begins to heal. The nicotine stains on your teeth and fingers will slowly go away, and your lungs will begin to repair themselves. You may still have other health effects from smoking, but your blood will begin to circulate better and you will have a much healthier complexion overall. Quitting smoking is one of the best things that you can do to stay youthful, so if this happens to be one of your vices, start your journey to quitting smoking today!

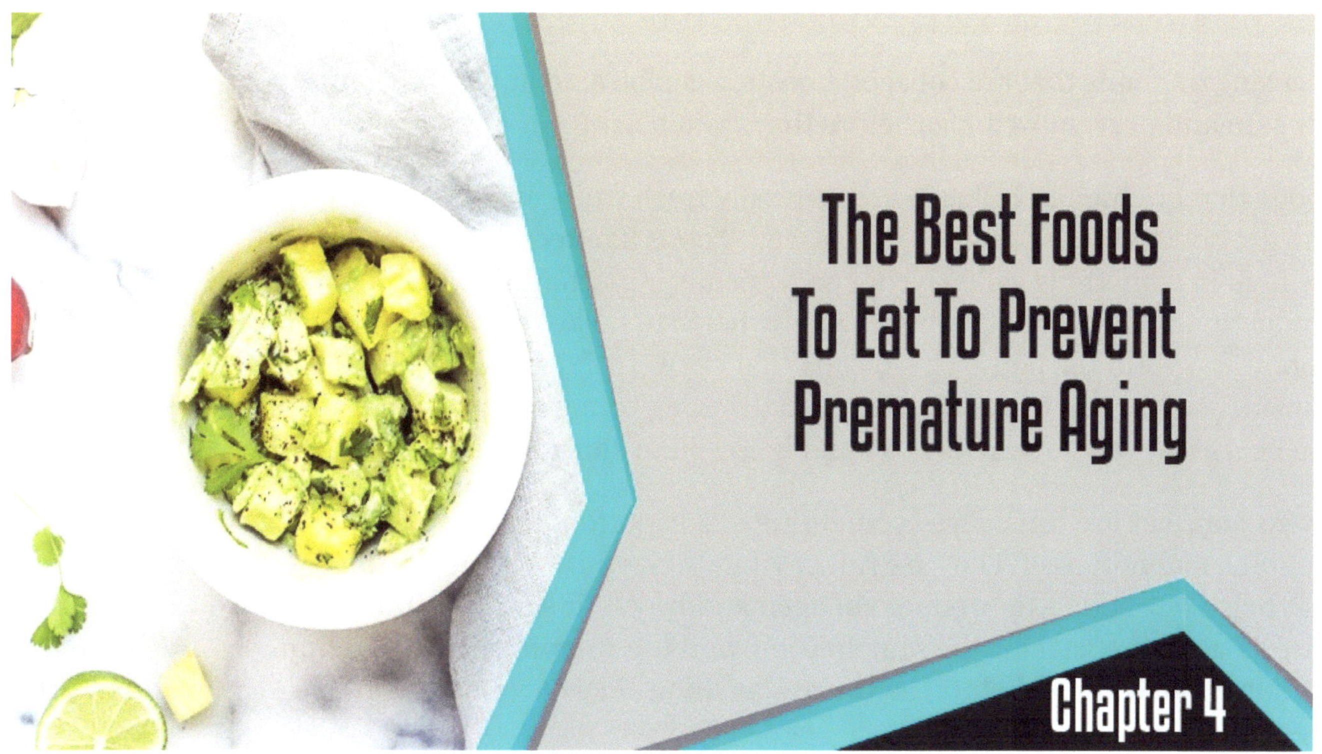

The Best Foods to Eat To Prevent Premature Aging

It is no secret that the key to a healthy lifestyle is a good diet and exercise, but are there specific foods that can help us to maintain our most youthful appearance?

Yes! Looking and feeling great starts with eating the right foods, and there are some superfoods that specifically target the skin and help to enhance its elasticity and build collagen, allowing us to combat wrinkles and look exuberant!

For example, the phytonutrients that are contained in spinach can actually help us to prevent damage to the skin, particularly the type of damage that can be caused through too much exposure to the sun. Spinach contains lutein and beta-carotene, which are essential in helping our bodies to keep our skin flexible and improve elasticity. It's best to eat spinach fresh, rather than from the can, and to get the best benefits from it do your best not to overcook it, or simply enjoy it raw in your salads with other delicious garnishes that can also be great for the skin.

Integrating kale into your salads also wouldn't hurt. Kale is chock full of vitamin C, which can help us to boost our immune systems and make the processes in our bodies work well and synthesize collagen. Dark, leafy green vegetables also provide our bodies with vitamin A, which is also useful in boosting collagen levels.

Foods that are helpful in producing collagen production are particularly helpful in anti-aging practices. Collagen is a protein that our bodies naturally produce to maintain the elasticity and strength of our skin. When we are eating collagen boosting foods, it can have a positive impact on our bodies and help us to look as radiant as possible.

Focusing on foods that are collagen boosters can be a great way to reinforce the elasticity of our skin and prevent wrinkles before they even begin!

Foods that are high in collagen are generally fresh fruits and vegetables. However, you can also get boosted collagen from fish as well. Foods like red bell peppers and roasted tomatoes are high in something called lycopene, which is important in helping to boost collagen production and vitamin C, which actually helps to make the process of collagen building smoother within the body. This means that citrus fruits are also beneficial in preventing aging. Consider waking up in the morning and drinking some water with a little bit of lemon juice! It can be a great way to start the day and help you to stay focused on your hydration.

Sweet potatoes are considered something of a superfood because of their abundance of vitamins and minerals. They are full of vitamin A, which we mentioined earlier is something that helps our bodies to produce collagen and keep our skin youthful and improves elasticity. Carrots are beneficial for the same reason, and the rumors of carrots helping with eyesight are actually true, which is helpful as you age as things like our muscle and our sight begin to suffer over time.

Garlic has been touted for centuries as a great homeopathic way to keep the body healthy and balanced, and there is definitely something to it. Garlic is beneficial for the body in many ways, so including it in your diet is a great way to help yourself prevent aging. It contains the chemical taurine, which helps to build collagen and keep it strong.

Another superfood is avocado. Avocados are high in healthy fats and omega 3 fatty acids, which help us to keep our minds focused and concentrating on the things that are the most important to us. Not only does it improve our concentration and help us keep our minds healthy, but omega 3 fatty acids also contributes to collagen production as well! Avocados are versatile and delicious, and a good option for keeping our skin, hair, and even our fingernails looking vibrant and youthful!

Nuts, beans, seeds, and other sources of protein are also beneficial to our bodies. They are full of essential vitamins and minerals that reinforce our body's natural processes and help us to keep things moving along. Everything in our body needs certain vitamins and minerals to fuel them and do everything necessary to keep us healthy. Making sure we are consuming the foods that help our bodies to do their jobs the most efficiently is essential in keeping us youthful and combatting aging!

If you're feeling a little discouraged by having to eat mainly fruits and vegetables for their anti-aging properties, don't worry! There is a bright side. Dark chocolate is actually a great food for preventing aging and remaining youthful. Some people even claim that it can help us to reverse the results of aging in our bodies. When we are dealing with inflammation and stress, it can speed up the effects of aging.

Another useful thing to include in your diet for anti-aging is food that has been fermented. Fermented foods are full of probiotics and other important vitamins and minerals that help us to support gut health. When we aren't digesting things properly, we are not receiving the full extent of vitamins and minerals that we would typically be able to absorb. Having an imbalance in our stomachs can also give us gastrointestinal issues that can cause us pain and discomfort.

Fortunately, dark chocolate not only tastes delicious, but it can also help us to relieve inflammation. Not only that, but difficulties recalling information can also be combated by dark chocolate, along with anxiety. Stress can actually increase the speed of aging in our bodies, as will be covered in a later chapter, so using stress-relief techniques and eating dark chocolate can actually add years on to your life and improve your appearance! Who knew that chocolate could be so good for us?

Maintaining our bodies is the most important thing that we can do to prevent aging. As we get older, our bodies begin to slow down and they take more maintenance. If we aren't giving our bodies the vitamins and nutrients and minerals that they require to stay healthy then maintaining the body is almost impossible. There will be deficits, and sometimes even malnutrition. More likely than not, though, we will have chronic issues that develop over time because we are not keeping our bodies supplied with the nutrients they need to thrive. If you want to focus on anti-aging, the most effective way to do so is to examine your diet and stay active! Eating well will provide our bodies with everything they need to combat aging and remain youthful for the long haul.

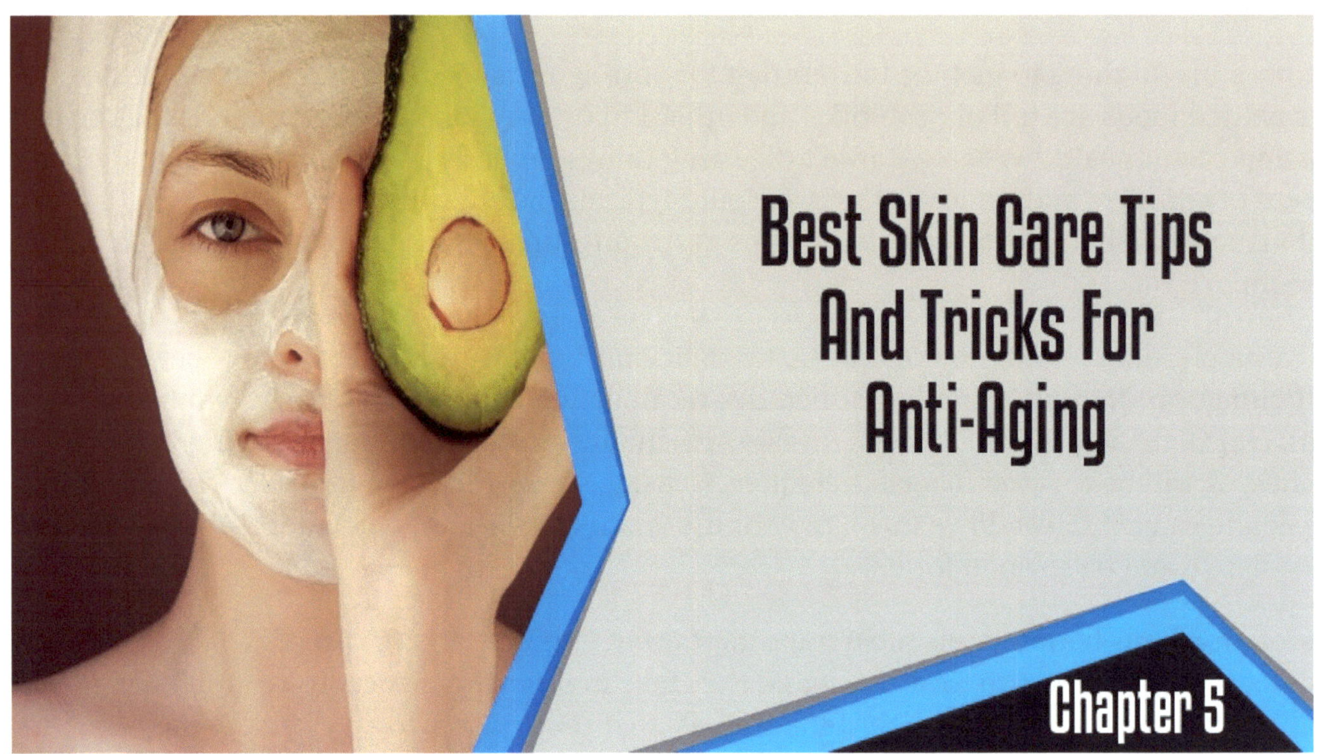

Best Skin Care Tips and Tricks for Anti-Aging

As mentioned in the beginning of the book, skin care is one of the most important things that we should focus on if we want to remain youthful and combat aging. Our skin is one of the most visible parts of our bodies and if we are not being mindful of it, then we will surely show signs of aging more than we would if we learned more about how to care for the skin and allow our bodies to thrive.

Fish oil capsules contain the omega 3 fatty acids that promote collagen production and keep our skin hydrated. When our skin's elasticity is promoted, wrinkles and other skin blemishes such as age spots and stretchmarks are far less likely! Avocado and eating the collagen promoting foods mentioned in a previous chapter are other great keys in improving our skin care and ensuring that our bodies are producing and utilizing collagen in a way that will help us to remain appearing as youthful as possible.

Another trick we already mentioned was using sunscreen and keeping the skin hydrated and protected from the sun's UV rays. Staying indoors or in shaded areas during the most sunny parts of the day can help us to avoid the harmful effects of the sun and allow us to maintain our skin's natural elasticity without drying it out or exposing it to the ultraviolet rays that can potentially cause cancer.

Something else that we can do is speak with a dermatologist about the different creams and treatments that we might be able to utilize to keep our skin healthy. Keeping the skin clean and hydrated can go a very long way in helping us to maintain a youthful appearance. It can also help us to stay healthier and to ensure that we are getting rid of toxins in our bodies rather than allowing them to linger.

When you are looking into a skin care regime, you will want to look into things that have derivatives of vitamin A, called retinoids. You should also stay on the lookout for antioxidants, peptides, hyaluronic acid, ceramids, and things that contain shea butter. Shea butter is one of the most hydrating of the compounds available and can be essential in keeping our skin hydrated and bright. It can also make the skin remarkably soft and smooth, and it smells good, too!

When it comes to our skin care, it can also be incredibly beneficial to remember that any time we sweat, we are releasing toxins and free radicals onto the surface of our skin. These things can cause bacteria and breakouts on our faces and bodies, so if you find yourself sweating, do everything in your power to shower it off as soon as possible afterward. It's important to maintain your skin's integrity and keep it clean.

However, after your showers, be sure that you moisturize. Put lotion onto your body afterward. You can also consider the option of air drying rather than drying off with a towel to enhance the hydration of your skin and protect your skin from the abrasion of your towel. Many people swear by air drying.

Something else you can do, while on the topic of showers, is to use cool water. Hot water can actually damage the skin and dry it out. however, using cool water, or at least as cool as you can stand it, is less likely to damage and dry the skin out. On top of that, it enhances the shine of our hair and protects the natural oils that our bodies produce to provide our hair with a beautiful sheen. If you suffer from dandruff or dry scalp, using cool water to wash and rinse your hair if nothing else can really work wonders!

Staying youthful is a full-time job and being able to develop a routine is one of the most important elements of maintaining our ability to utilize anti-aging techniques. Learn what products you want to use the most and avoid harsh scrubs that might cause abrasions to the skin. Once you know the best routine that works for you, turn it into a daily habit. It will only take a few minutes out of your day, but it will affect your skin for the better for the rest of your life. It's worth it! Determine your personal skin care routine and start to implement it today!

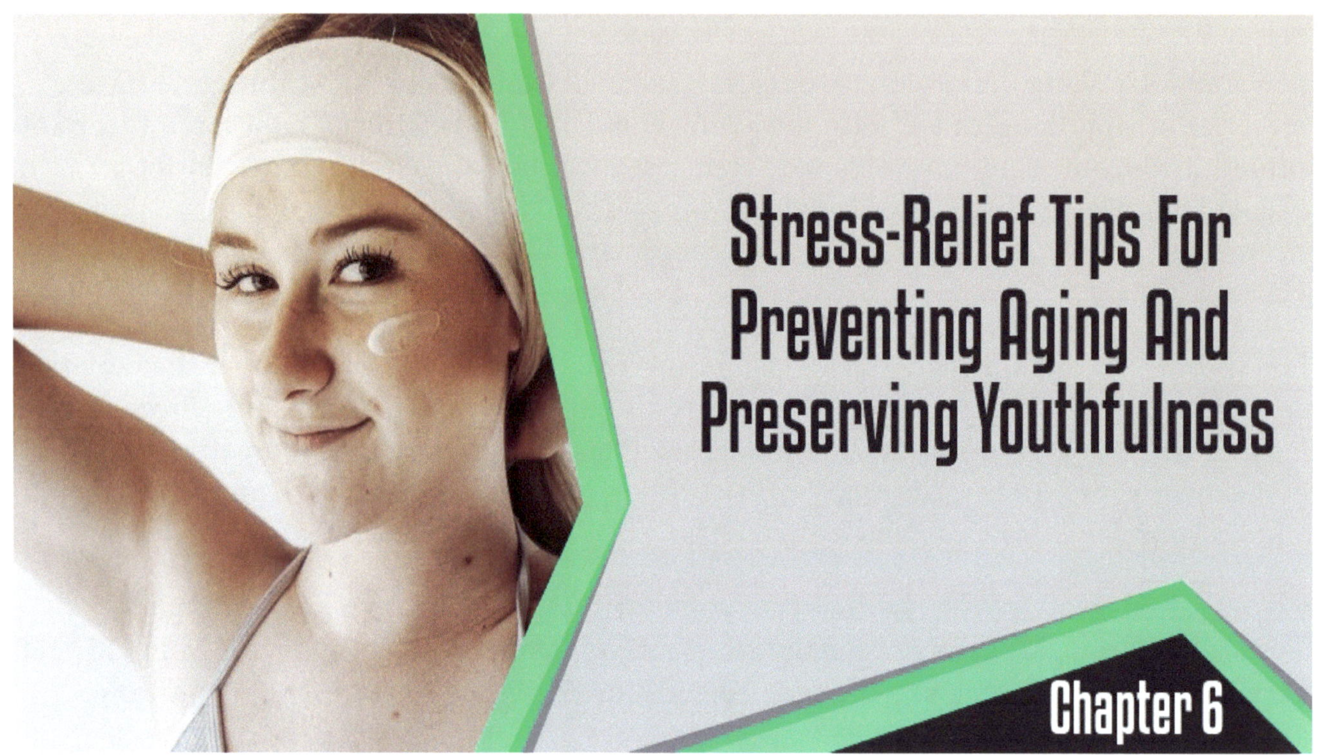

Stress-Relief Tips for Preventing Aging and Preserving Youthfulness

Stress is bad enough but understanding the way that stress can negatively impact the body can actually make us feel stressed about stress! It's a horrible cycle, and nobody wins. Forget the wrinkles that we get from making faces when we are feeling anxious, what about the way that our bodies begin to produce cortisol when we are feeling overwhelmed? What about the way that heightened cortisol levels can lead to decreases in bone density and muscle mass? What about the way that heightened cortisol levels can cause heart problems and diabetes, or a related issue in hypoglycemia?

Yeah, wrinkles are a huge side effect, but that's nowhere near as important as realizing just how potent a killer stress can be. And it kills us silently. There is nothing more important than our health, so learning how to destress can actually be one of the most crucial things that we can do in order to thrive and maintain a healthy and youthful lifestyle.

Have you ever watched children as they interact with the world? Would you say that they tend to be stressed out and prone to bad moods? No, usually children have a tendency to live in the moment and they don't let their stresses bog them down. Instead of wondering what they should have done differently and letting themselves become overwhelmed by the possibilities and their mistakes, instead, they have a mindset of trying to figure out what to do next. They are proactive and thoughtful, but they don't dwell in the negativity the same way as adults do.

Of course, that is a generalization, but consider the lesson here. Rather than dwelling in the things that we can't control and things that have already been said and done, it is time to be proactive. It is time to think about what we can do to move forward. It's also important that we allow ourselves to have fun and to prioritize the things that actually make us feel happy.

That's not to say it's more important to play and have fun than it is to pay the bills and work. It simply means that learning the ways that you relax and enjoy the moment can be crucial in the maintenance of our mental and physical health. If you feel overwhelmed and stressed out, or find yourself suffering from the famous, "all work and no play" syndrome, take a moment to think about what it is that makes you feel good and how you can begin to implement things into your life that make you happier.

Something that can help a lot of people with stress is physical activity. Naturally boosting our serotonin levels with exercise and movement can be incredibly helpful and give us mood-enhancing chemicals without even needing to take a prescription antidepressant. Not only that, but we feel good when we exercise because we know that we are doing something important for our bodies to help us look and feel great. It is a good way to help us boost our confidence and feel the best way about us possible. We will discuss physical exercise and its correlations with anti-aging later in this book!

Another common way that people attempt to battle stress in their daily lives is meditation. Mindfulness meditation is perhaps one of the most effective methods of meditation for people who want to be able to slow down in their lives and pay attention to the little things. It can help us to remember to live in the moment rather than getting lost in our heads, and ultimately taking at least five minutes out of our day to practice meditation can significantly reduce our stress levels and help us to live our best lives possible.

Another thing that can help with stress is to speak with a counselor or therapist. Many people think of it as a bad thing, but sometimes it can be nice to have an objective party around who is willing to listen to our problems and help us to work through them in a constructive way. Sometimes we accumulate stress that we don't even realize or acknowledge because they are related to issues that have been affecting us since our developmental stages or childhood traumas. While we may be living to the best of our ability, there is always something worthwhile about taking the time out to be introspective and learn more about ourselves so that we can navigate the world in the most effective way possible.

Whether you consider therapy or not, journaling and writing down the things that bother you can be a good way to process your feelings and events that are happening and stay focused on the present moment. It is good to express yourself and to keep in mind the fact that when we don't express the things that bother us, they can often build up until they create situations in our lives that are beyond our control at that point. Rather than letting your unconscious energies dictate the way you live your life, acknowledge them in a way that makes it possible for you to move on and stay focused on the next step in making your life better and accomplishing your goals!

Something else that can help us to reduce stress is to stop or slow down our intake of caffeine. This will not only help us to stop feeling anxious, but it will help our blood vessels to expand rather than restrict the flow of blood and improve our circulation, which is hugely beneficial for those who want to remain youthful and slow the effects of aging. It can be difficult to do, but there are other ways to get your energy levels up in the morning, such as through exercise and drinking water with lemon in it for a nice boost of citrus and energizing vitamin C. You can also take B-complex vitamins for a burst of natural energy that will ultimately help your body to function and thrive!

Don't let stress be the silent killer that is preventing you from becoming the person you most want to be. It can begin to show on our faces and affect our health, so if you want to live a happy and youthful life, you have to make sure that you are feeling happy and youthful! Follow these tips to begin working on reducing your stress levels and naturally enabling your body to do its own anti-aging process, starting now!

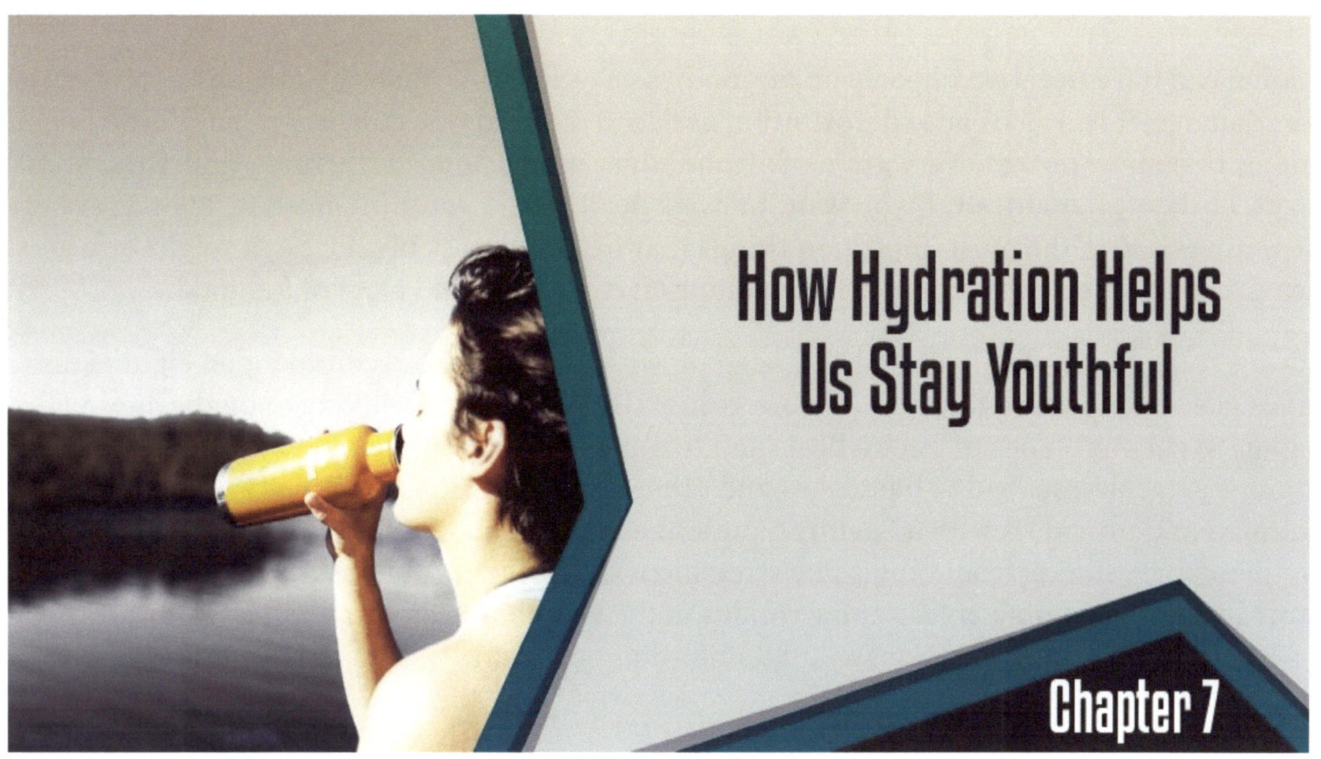

How Hydration Helps Us Stay Youthful

It can't be stressed enough just how important it is to keep our bodies hydrated. When we are dehydrated it can cause a plethora of issues within the body, including thickening of the blood, inefficient removal of toxins and waste products, and even heart palpitations and other scary issues. Not only that but going only three days without water can cause us to die, and there is sufficient evidence to state that a large portion of the population is dehydrated a majority of the time. So many people quench their thirsts with sugary drinks that can actually do us more harm than good. Sugar is one of the most dangerous things that we can put into our bodies in large quantities, so it is important to stay aware of what we are drinking.

It may surprise you to realize that even drinking juices is not as healthy for you as drinking water is. Fruit juice doesn't contain the same amount of fiber that eating an actual fruit does, which means that we are mainly consuming natural sugars and a few vitamins without the full benefit of eating the fruit. It will not help us to eliminate toxins the same way eating a whole piece of fruit would, and it can overload our body with sugars. Whether they are natural sugars or not, too much sugar in our bodies can lead to weight gain and the destruction of important cells. It can make it difficult for us to concentrate and lead to a mind fog, along with a slew of other possible problems down the line, including diabetes.

Another issue that people have when they reach for a cool beverage is that they tend to want to drink things that contain caffeine or alcohol. Caffeine is also dangerous for our bodies. It can restrict the blood flow and it actually has a tendency to dehydrate us rather than to hydrate us. Sure, you can drink it and stop feeling thirsty, but it doesn't provide our bodies with the necessary hydration. It can also leave us feeling a little bit sluggish and we can suffer from caffeine crashes as well.

Alcohol can have negative impacts on our bodies as well. Other than the obvious potential for liver damage, it can also cause dehydration and lead to dried out skin. There have even been studies that show us that every gram of alcohol that we consume can actually cause the brain to age 11 days prematurely. If you want to live a healthy and youthful lifestyle, taking care of the brain is one of the most important things that we could possibly do. So, it might be a good idea to cut down or even cut out the consumption of caffeine and alcohol for good.

However, if you can stay hydrated and keep up with drinking the recommended eight eight-ounce glasses of water daily, then you are going to look radiant. Drinking enough water will help us to rid our bodies of free radicals and toxins that might otherwise compromise our immune systems and lead to blemishes and other issues. It will also help us to keep our skin hydrated and provide it with a healthy glow and a nice plump texture. You will have a lower likelihood of suffering from things like stretchmarks or other problems that can happen when our skin is dry. Avoiding cracks and wrinkles in the skin may seem impossible, but in reality, it is within our abilities, as long as we are doing what our bodies need us to do and consuming enough water!

It can seem difficult to get the right amount of water. It just doesn't always taste good and it can be difficult to crave something that doesn't seem to have much of a flavor. However, there are many ways that you can spice your water up so that it isn't quite as difficult to drink it. For example, you could try to put pitchers of water in your refrigerator that contain berries, other fruits, or even cucumbers. Having cold, naturally flavored water readily available to you can be an incredible and delicious way to up your water intake and cut down on unhealthy sugars and artificial sodas or alcohol.

There are also flavoring packets available in most grocery stores. Many of them are sugar free and have a good variety of flavor. Using them can be a good way to help you to break your dependence on soda or other artificial drinks while providing flavor and sweetness and allowing you to drink as much water daily as is required for your body to function to its highest potential.

We can also do our best to turn our water intake into a routine. Eight eight-ounce bottles of water can translate roughly to about four bottles of water daily at minimum, depending on the size of the bottle. If we wake up, determined to drink a bottle of water before and during breakfast, a bottle and a half between then and lunch, and a bottle with and after dinner, then it can actually be pretty easy for us to begin to get the recommended water intake.

Another thing that we can do to drink more water is to download an application on our cell phones that will help us to track our water intake. When we do this, we set a goal for ourselves daily and are able to track it and make sure that we are getting enough of the most important fluid. Some of the apps out there will provide you with little rewards for being able to meet your goals. It can make it a fun and helpful experience to drink our water and make sure that we are doing everything possible to maintain our health and make choices that will help us to stay youthful and healthy.

Overall, drinking water can help us in just about every way imaginable, and on top of that, it can make our skin radiant, soft, and pleasant. If we want to avoid the issues associated with dried out skin that lacks elasticity, then an easy solution is to simply ensure that we are getting enough water on a daily basis.

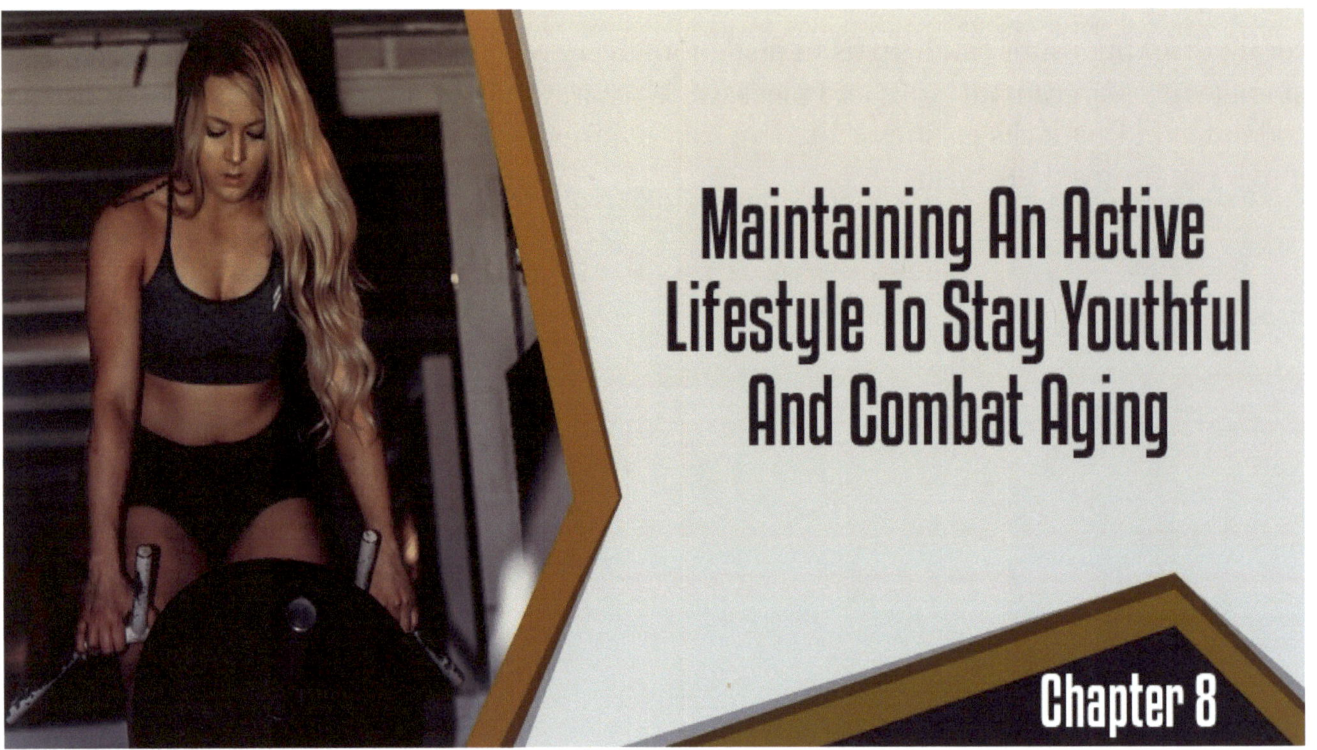

Maintaining an Active Lifestyle to Stay Youthful and Combat Aging

Anybody who wants to maintain a youthful appearance and reduce the signs of aging should take into consideration their lifestyle. Are you active? Do you spend a majority of your time in your chair at home watching television or browsing the internet? What do you enjoy doing that you know for sure is good for your body? How much exercise do you get daily? Weekly? Monthly?

If you ask yourself these things and you realize that you may not be getting enough activity during your daily lives, have no fear. All of us have our strengths and weaknesses, and it can be easy to fall into a routine that lacks more activity than what we need to do to get through our daily lives. All of us have the power to change our routines and do exercises that will help us to maintain our flexibility and keep our bodies active and in their prime.

I'm not saying that we all must be yoga gurus by the age of fifty. The truth is that not all of us are going to be at the same level of fitness or even capable of the same types of exercise. Sometimes, simply lifting your legs off the ground in repetitions can be just as good for you as running a lap, depending on who you are and what situation you are in.

What should happen, rather than pressuring yourself into launching into an exercise routine that could end up hurting you or lowering your self-esteem because you haven't properly built up to it, is you should have a conversation with your doctor about the kind of exercises that would most benefit you. When you learn what you should be doing and how often you should be doing it, then simply begin to make it a part of your daily routine.

If you are told that you don't have to restrict your exercise, then you should still probably start slow as your body is getting used to the new workout and allow yourself to get acclimated to the change in your routine. It can be discouraging to throw ourselves into a new activity that our bodies are not ready for only to find out that we can't keep up with the ambitious pace that we set for ourselves.

Instead, start slow but stay consistent. Do one thing every day until it feels natural, and then add in something else until you have a whole new routine set up. Make sure you are comfortable with the exercises you have chosen, and if possible, try to find activities that don't necessarily feel like work to you.

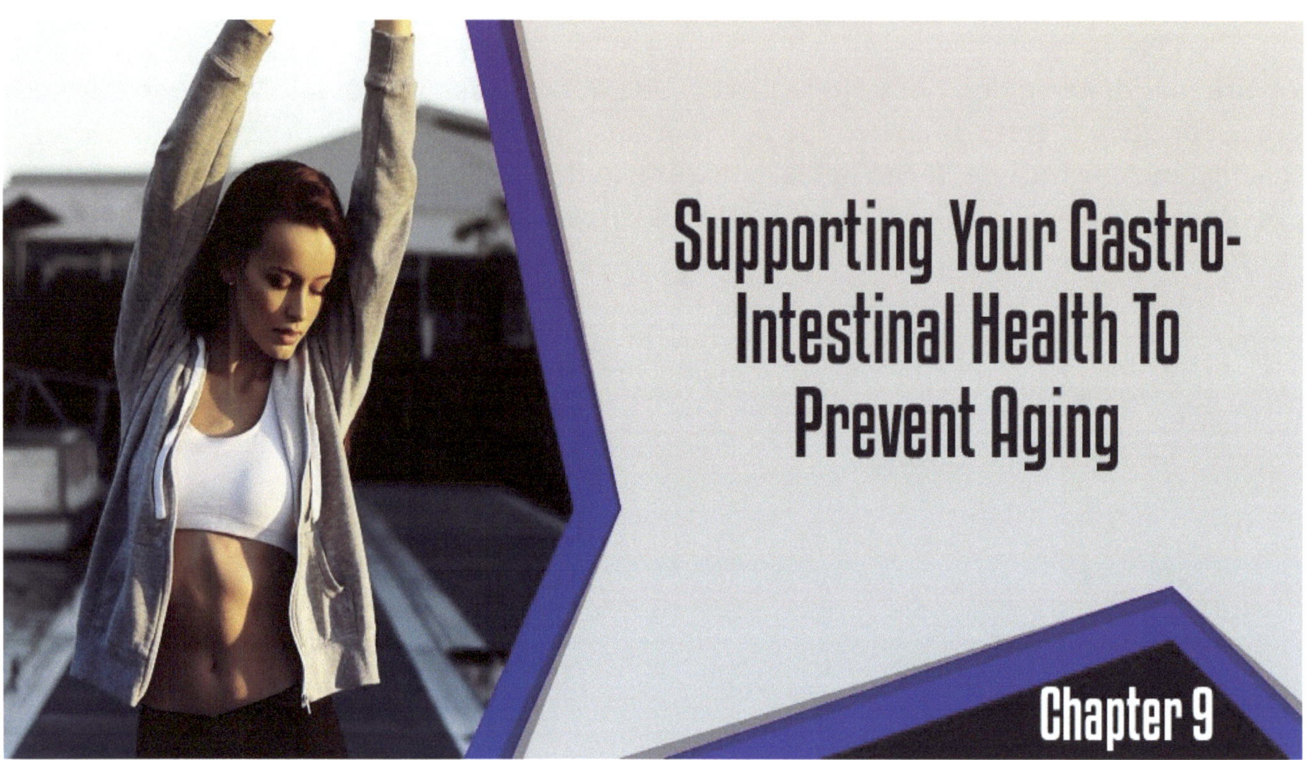

Supporting Your Gastro-Intestinal Health to Prevent Aging

The older we get, the less responsive certain areas of our bodies become. One examples of this is our stomachs. Our gastrointestinal tracts are a delicate system that helps our bodies to maintain balance. If our bodies become too acidic or too alkaline, it can have different effects. Generally, a balance is a good thing, and making sure that we have the right bacteria working for us in our guts is a very important thing.

As we age, it can become more common to have issues with digestion. We may not be able to eat certain foods that we used to because now they no longer agree with us. When we eat an unhealthy diet, we can suffer from inflammation which can contribute to intestinal distress. One of the most important things that we can do to combat this is to focus on ensuring that we are providing our intestinal tract with the good bacteria that it needs to help us thrive and prevent disease.

So what can we do about it?

As mentioned earlier in the book, we can do our best to integrate foods that have been fermented. Fermented cabbage called kimchi is particularly common in the Korean marketplace and has been utilized for centuries to ensure a healthy digestive system and prolonged good health.

When we live on the Standard American Diet (also appropriately known as the SAD diet), we are eating foods that cause a huge amount of inflammation within our bodies. The bacteria in our guts can play a massive role in the way our bodies function. It can affect our brain function, our metabolism, and even the way our immune systems respond to dangers to our system.

If we are not creating a healthy environment and killing the good bacteria and replacing them with bad, then we are going to end up feeling awful and not even being able to put our fingers on why or how we aren't feeling right.

Fortunately, we can address these things and make sure that the foods we are eating are actually supportive of our gut health rather than diminishing of it. When we know how important it is to avoid inflammation, it is far easier to stay motivated to make conscious choices about what we put in our bodies. When we have issues with inflammation in our intestines it can lead to some really ugly problems, such as inflammatory bowel disease. This can cause upset stomachs and gastrointestinal discomfort that can sometimes be embarrassing and difficult to control.

However, the more we know about how to treat our bodies and why, the better off we are in creating a body and lifestyle that will support us in remaining youthful and feeling and looking great! So how can you support your gastrointestinal health? You can easily find probiotics at your local pharmacies, along with food and drinks that contain probiotics that are good for your health and will help to balance out the bad bacteria in your intestines with the good. May foods also contain probiotics, such as yogurt, and, as mentioned before, fermented foods.

Don't dismiss the importance of your gastrointestinal health. The more inflammation there is in our bodies the more uncomfortable we are and the less active we will want to be. But being active is one of the keys to leading a healthy and youthful life, so by putting your body first you are paving the way to living your best life possible!

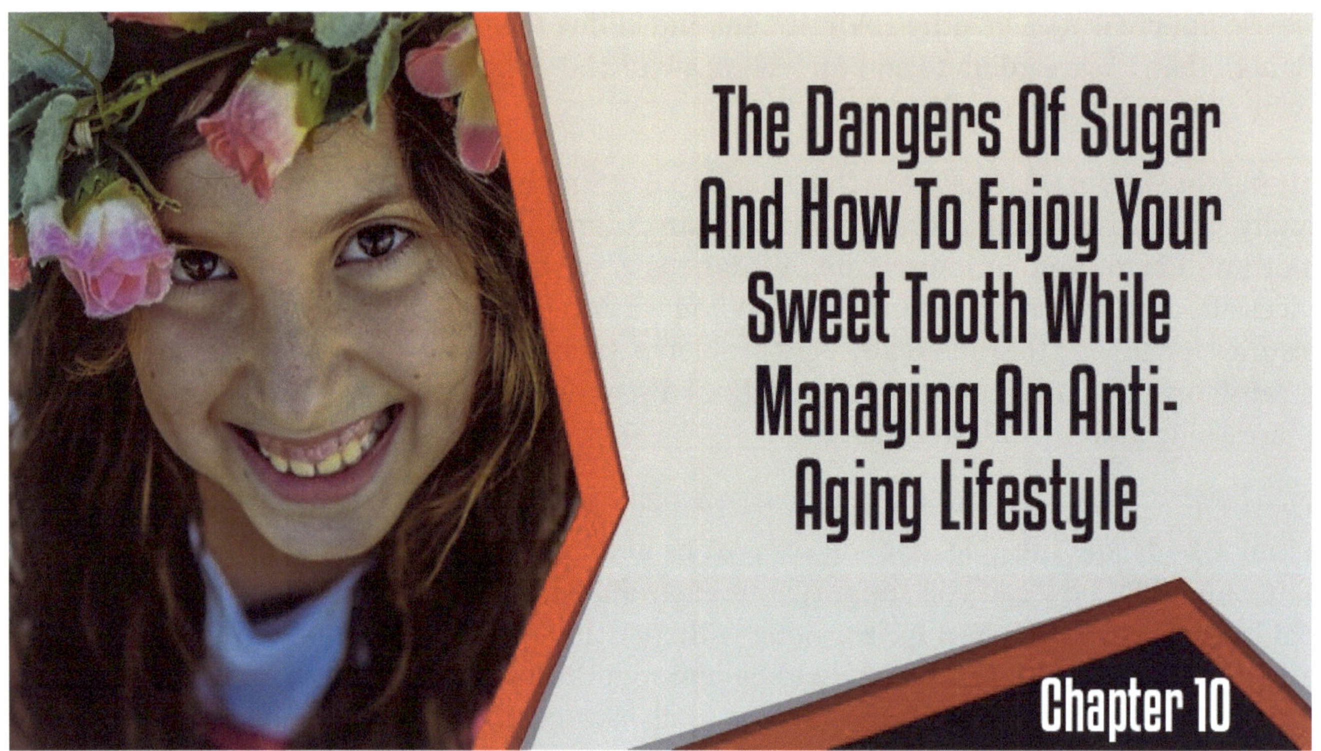

The Dangers of Sugar and How to Enjoy Your Sweet Tooth While Managing an Anti-Aging Lifestyle

All of us enjoy a nice snack here and there, but the things that we choose to snack on can make a huge difference in the way our bodies begin to react to aging. In fact, some things can actually speed up the aging process and cause us to look older than we are prematurely. It's important to identify these things and try our best to address them in our lifestyles.

Sugar, for example, is extremely bad for us. Specifically, processed and refined sugar. Natural sugar isn't anywhere near as bad for our bodies unless we are diabetic and should be avoiding sugar completely or keeping an eye on our sugar intake in general.

Unfortunately, typical refined sugars such as what we would find in bags for sale in our local grocery stores are chock full of glucose and fructose. These things actually have a bad reaction with the collagen that our bodies produce and can ultimately deteriorate them, which can cause our skin to lose its elasticity. When we eat too much sugar, we can develop dark spots on our skin, have a more difficult time healing our bodies when they are injured, and we are prone to skin issues. Eating too much sugar can give us blemishes, wrinkles, and a tightness in the skin, which can cause it to appear more stiff and rigid and lack in moisture and the supple smoothness most people associate with youth.

Some have compared the interaction that our collagen building cells have to sugar as the way that a banana begins to brown when it is left out for a while. There is a chemical reaction between them that triggers entropy, and ultimately it makes it more difficult for us to build the important cells that help us to maintain our healthy and youthful appearance. That isn't even going into the way that it can cause excessive weight gain, which can seriously diminish our health and ability to appear youthful. The worse off our bodies are the more difficult it is for us to remain looking and feeling youthful.

Sugar can damage our skin because of something called glycation. When we eat an abundance of sugar, the sugar that gets in our bloodstream ends up bonding with the healthier proteins in our skin that are related to collagen production. When this reaction takes place, our blood fills with something known as advanced glycation end products, appropriately known as AGEs. When our blood is overpowered by these things, the good proteins are damaged and our skin suffers as a result, making positive collagen formation difficult, if not impossible, to occur, and leaving our skin more brittle, dry, and less elastic.

Sugar can also make it difficult for the body's natural antioxidants to thrive. These enzymes are crucial in helping us to get rid of the toxins in our bodies and free our bloodstream from the free radicals that can move up to our brain to cause issues, sometimes even becoming as extreme as dementia. If we aren't able to properly get rid of the waste products in our bodies, then not only will our appearance suffer, but our overall health will as well. Our immune systems will not be as strong and we will have a difficult time properly oxidizing our blood, which can affect all our organs in the long run. We may even suffer from hormonal imbalances, which, as we all know, is already something that our bodies struggle with as time goes on and would best be avoided if and when possible.

If you are concerned that sugar may have begun to affect your body negatively, there are some signs that your sugar intake may be compromising your health and youthfulness. If your skin is discolored or abnormally red in some places, if your skin looks shiny and hard rather than soft and smooth, if you have lines around your top lip, if your neck area sags, and if you find that when you laugh, deeper crevices than normal appear, then it is highly possible that you are feeling the results of the consumption of too much sugar and that it is already chemically altering your body and making it difficult for you to naturally combat the signs of aging.

Anti-aging is a delicate process, and one that is best done with the removal of processed sugars from the diet. You could attempt to eat them in moderation, but don't be surprised when you end up simply craving more and more of it. This is because processed sugars are actually highly addicting, and we can have physical withdrawals if we start to eat it and then stop abruptly. It is better to cut out sugar entirely than it is to try and eat processed and refined sugars in moderation, because they can be so physically addicting that the cycle becomes very difficult to break, if not impossible.

Fortunately, there are some solutions if you find that you have a sweet tooth. Natural sugars can be found in fruits and having fruits as a snack can be a great way to help us to stay on a path of anti-aging. The natural vitamins and minerals in fruit along with their collagen producing effects can really keep our skin vibrant and our bodies full of energy.

Drinking a lot of water is another great way to help us to repair the effects of too much sugar intake. There are some tips in previous chapters on how to increase water intake if that is something that you struggle with. It is also important, if not crucial, to scrutinize the products that you are putting into your body. High fructose corn syrup is a major factor in the aging process, as it is pure sugar in liquid form and it is found in many, many processed foods, snacks, and beverages. Make sure that you are avoiding it at all costs to ensure that you are allowing your body the chance to purge the bad things and build healthy collagen proteins.

Detoxing the skin and the body is another good way to reverse the effects of sugar on the skin. There are several different methods to do this and it would be best to consult your doctor or primary care physician about what route is the best for you to take, as all our bodies are different and respond differently to different treatments. Another thing to do is to take supplements for B-complex, as it will help our bodies to get rid of the bad and maintain the good. B1 and B6 in particular are helpful in combatting the signs of aging due to a diet that is excessive in sugar.

You could also try to use sugar that isn't as processed and refined, such as natural cane sugars. These sugars are a little bit easier for our bodies to break down because they are concentrated from the natural sugars produced by sugar cane plants. When we utilize sugars that are natural and easier for our bodies to digest, they aren't quite as destructive as the refined sugars found in other products. If you want to live a life of anti-aging, finding a compromise between sweets and what will actually help us to remain youthful can be incredibly important.

There is also the option of replacing the snacks and desserts that you love that are full of processed and refined sugars with snacks and desserts that are full of natural sugars instead. And by this we don't mean getting rid of cakes and brownies. Rather, consider looking into a raw food cookbook. Raw food diets are not for everybody, but they can offer incredible and healthy alternatives to refined sugar-filled desserts that instead use things like dates, nuts, and agave nectar or honey as a way to keep things sweet and support our health rather than by harming it. Rather than eating a chocolate pudding in a plastic container or making it from a powder full of processed chemicals and sugar, you could use a food processor to create a pudding that is just as rich and sweet using avocado, cocoa powder, and a natural sweetener of your choice! Some of these recipes are so simple it seems almost impossible, but they exist and they are incredible resources for those who have a sweet tooth but who know that refined sugars are slowly destroying our bodies.

However, you choose to approach this information, knowing that eating an excessive amount of refined sugar is important. There are solutions, and there are ways that we can begin to repair the damages that have already been done. Knowledge is power, and we can keep taking steps forward for our health, starting now!

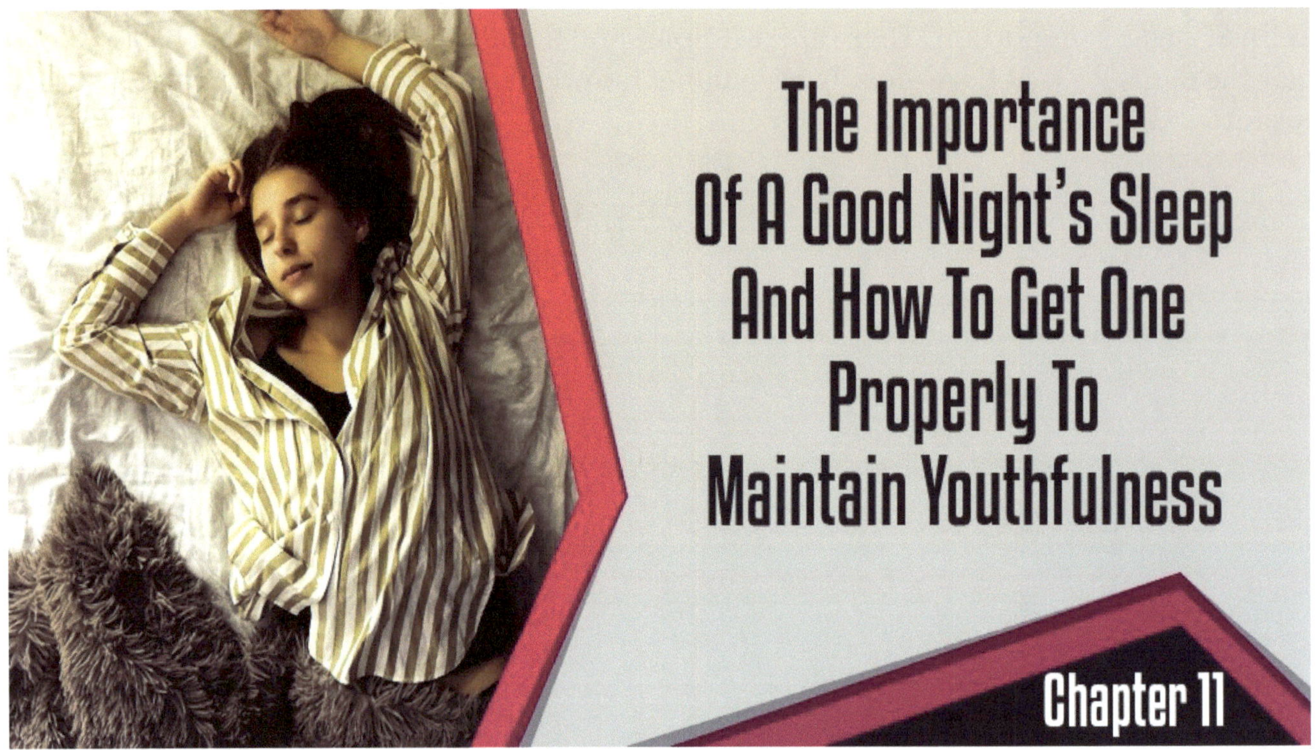

The Importanced of a Good Night's Sleep and How to Get One Properly to Maintain Youthfulness

Have you ever heard the phrase, "I need to get my beauty sleep?" Have you ever used it? Well, you should! Getting enough sleep is probably one of the most important ways that we can maintain our appearance and continue our lives feeling energized and bringing a youthful energy to everything that we do. Every time we neglect our sleeping schedules, we are making our lives more difficult and robbing our bodies of the rest that they need to maintain a youthful appearance.

However, there are some caveats to this. While ten hours of beauty sleep is recommended, you have to be conscientious about how you sleep. When we sleep on our sides or keep our faces on our pillows, it increases the occurrence of fine lines. One of the ways to combat this is to try to get comfortable with the idea of sleeping on our backs. Another thing that we can do is to switch out our pillowcases and spend a little money on a higher thread count or silk so that the fine lines that occur in our sleep are less likely to form.

A lot of people have a hard time getting and maintaining a good sleep. If you have a hard time falling asleep, consider whether or not you ingest a good amount of caffeine during the day. Maybe you could consider switching to a decaf diet after noon or cutting yourself off of sugar and caffeine intake after a certain point in the day so that it's safely out of your system by the time it's time to lay down and get your beauty sleep.

You might also benefit from a noise machine during the night, or a soothing ritual of nice scents diffused to help you relax and enjoy a peaceful time before bed. You could also make sure that you are getting enough bright light during the day, like going out into the sun, but keep in mind that you don't want to expose your skin to the dangers of the sun's rays if possible and wear sunscreen if you use this method and keep your skin covered. On the topic of lights, at night, don't allow yourself to be exposed to too much blue light. This is the kind of light that we get from screens, such as from a computer or a phone screen.

This blue light emulates sunlight and it tricks our minds into thinking that it is still daylight out and that there is no reason to begin calming down and readying ourselves for a good night's rest.

There are blue light filters you can use on your phone and computer screens, and glasses that you can order that filter out blue light if you really have no choice but to work on your phone or computer in the evening.

Another helpful thing to do to get the best rest at night is to avoid napping during the day. This may seem like common sense, but it is worth noting. Sometimes we just don't rest well enough at night and we feel groggy and uncomfortable during the day, so a nap may seem like a good solution. Unfortunately, it just adds to the cycle of poor rest at night and a groggy day after. Break the cycle by toughing it through the grogginess and skipping the nap so your night's rest will be a higher quality!

Using these tips and tricks should help you to maintain a regular sleeping schedule and help your body to get the time that it needs to energize itself and help us to prevent signs of aging. When we rest well, we feel well, and we also look well as well! Say goodbye to the bags under your eyes and hello to a new life full of energy and vitality!

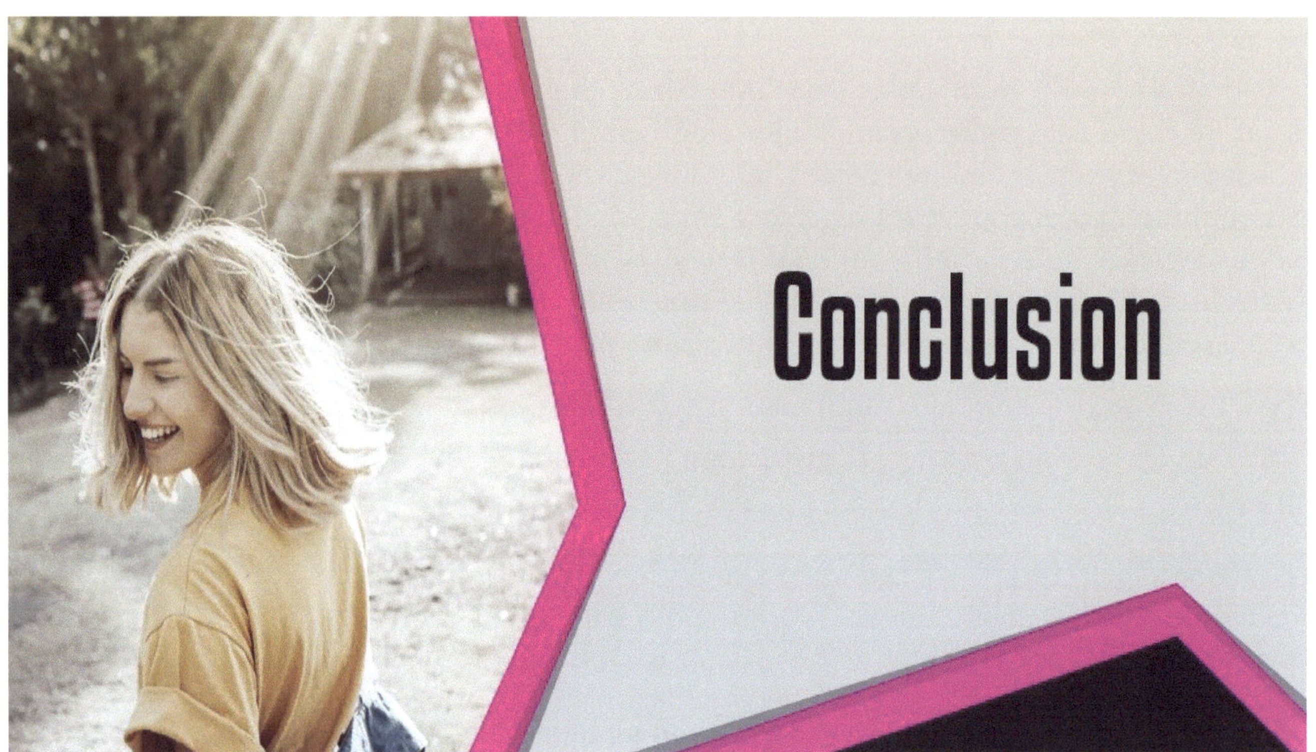

Conclusion

Our bodies are sensitive, even though they can make it through a lot. Many people assume that because they are still living day to day without huge issues that they are healthy, when that is not necessarily the case. It takes proper maintenance of our bodies before we are able to really utilize some of the natural splendor that they are capable of.

We can decrease signs of aging. We can maintain our bodies to function as well as they possibly can. But we can only do that if we are willing to pay attention to the things that we are doing and create a better routine that allows us to thrive. So many of us get comfortable in bad habits and routines that harm us rather than help us. We might not see right away how our bad habits will affect us in the future, but when the future shows up and we are seeing the results, it can be a little bit jarring.

Fortunately, this book is full of the advice and wisdom that you need to take control of your life and begin an anti-aging journey that will leave you looking and feeling better than ever! All you must do is take the first step and see for yourself the amazing results.

So, what are you waiting for? Ditch the sugar, take a walk around the block, wash your face, and get some rest! There is nothing stopping you except yourself, so do whatever you possibly can to give your body the care that it needs so that it can start to take care of you as well. This book has shown you how, so begin the anti-aging process today!

Anti-Aging - Cheat Sheet

The importance of taking care of your skin

- Skin shows the appearance of age
- There are three layers of skin.
- Epidermis contains keratin and lagerhans cells that protect the skin
- Signals from nerve endings travel from the skin to the brain
- The dermis regulates blood flow and temperature

Staying out of the sun for health's sake

- UV rays from the sun are dangerous
- Sun exposure can dry out the skin and cause wrinkles
- Sun exposure can cause cancer

Bad habits to avoid preventing aging and preserve youthfulness

- Don't rub your eyes
- Rubbing your eyes causes the skin to thin and look older
- Quit smoking
- Smoking has several health consequences including premature aging

The best foods to eat to prevent premature aging

- Foods that enhance collagen production are key
- Spinach
- Kale
- Sweet potatoes and carrots
- Garlic
- Avocado
- Dark chocolate
- Nuts, beans, and seeds

Best skin care tips and tricks for anti-aging

- Fish oil capsules

- Healthy diet
- Staying hydrated
- Look for skin care products containing retinoids, peptides, antioxidants, ceramids, and hyaluronic acid.
- Wash any time you sweat
- Consider air drying after showers
- Moisturize with lotion after showers

Stress-relief tips for preventing aging and preserving youthfulness

- Journaling
- Antidepressants
- Naturally boosting serotonin levels with exercise
- Meditation
- Counseling
- Reduce caffeine intake
- How hydration helps us stay youthful
- Water helps us remove waste products
- Dehydration thickens the blood, reduces toxin removal, and causes heart palpitations
- Juice is also unhealthy as it concentrates sugars that can damage the body
- Alcohol dehydrates the body and causes other health issues
- Drink eight, eight-ounce glasses of water daily
- Water detoxes the skin and keeps it looking radiant
- Water helps the organs to function and do their jobs efficiently
- Try tricks to drinking enough water, such as flavoring it naturally with fruit or cucumbers.

Maintaining an active lifestyle to stay youthful and combat aging

- All of us have different levels of physical activity
- Take it slow and stay in your comfort zone
- Make exercise a part of your daily routine

Supporting your gastro-intestinal health to prevent aging

- Stop eating the SAD diet
- Maintain good gut balance
- Probiotics in your food and supplements

Dangers of sugar and how to enjoy your sweet tooth while managing an anti-aging lifestyle

- Sugar can cause blemishes, wrinkles, tight skin
- Sugar prevents collagen building
- Sugar bonds with healthy proteins and fills blood with advanced glycation end products
- AGEs makes collagen production difficult and leaves skin brittle

Importance of sleep and how to get good rest

- Get at least ten hours of sleep
- Sleep on your back
- Use silk pillowcases
- Noise machines, avoiding caffeine, avoid blue light

About the Author

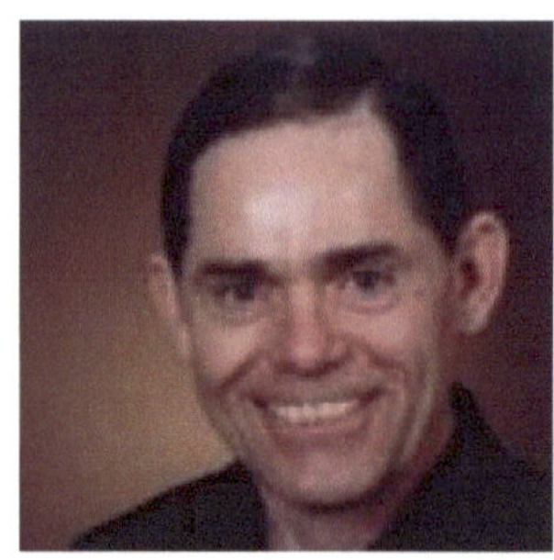

I am a published writer with numerous books on Amazon for Kindle and other publishing platforms … both in electronic and Print On Demand (POD) formats.

While most of my self-published books are on health and fitness in general, my topics of interest currently are more toward 1) aging baby boomers and the older population and 2) low content books, like word activity books, journals, planners and calendars.

Besides my own writing, I also ghostwrite eBooks, books, reports, articles, autoresponder series, blogs and Kindle conversions for my client base on a variety of topics. I'm currently using Microsoft's Office Suite including Word, PowerPoint and Publisher, along with Affinity Publisher and Designrr for writing and publishing.

Go to my website at http://ronknesswriting.com for more information or to request a quote: https://ronknesswriting.com/ghostwriting-quote-request-form.

For a complete list of my books published on Amazon, go to https://www.amazon.com/Ron-Kness/e/B0072M6PYO.